BASIC YOGA FOR EVERYBODY

B·A·S·I·C
YOGA
for
EVERYBODY

84 Cards with
Accompanying Handbook

GERTRUD HIRSCHI

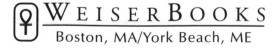

WEISERBOOKS
Boston, MA/York Beach, ME

First published in 1998 by
RED WHEEL/WEISER, LLC
368 Congress Street
Boston, MA 02210

Library of Congress Cataloging-in-Publication Data

Hirschi, Gertrud.
  [Lust auf Yoga. English]
  Basic Yoga for Everybody/ Gertrud Hirschi.
    p. cm.
  Translation of: Lust auf Yoga.
  Includes index.
  ISBN 1-57863-103-3 (paper : alk. paper)
  1. Yoga, Hatha. I. Title
RA781.7.H57513 1998
613.7'046--dc21   97-52599
                                                                       CIP

Translated by Christine M. Grimm
Book and cover design by Kathryn Sky-Peck
Illustrations by Ito Joyoatmojo

Typeset in 11 point Granjon

PRINTED AND BOUND IN HONG KONG BY C & C OFFSET PRINTING CO.

10 09 08 07 06 05 04 03 02
12 11 10 9 8 7 6 5 4

*The paper used in this publication meets the minimum requirements of the American
National Standard for Information Sciences—Permanence of Paper for
Printed Library Materials Z39.48–1992(R1997).*

CONTENTS

DEAR READER

When Karin Vial, editor at the Hermann Bauer Publishing Company in Germany, suggested that I design a yoga card set, I was immediately excited by the idea. I hope that the enthusiasm that constantly accompanied and inspired me as I created this card set will inspire you, too, when you work with these cards.

A person who buys cards doesn't want to first read a book, but wants to start right away with the "game." However, you should read chapters 2, 3, and 4 before you begin, since you can learn everything there that you need to know about using the cards. I've kept the instructions for working with yoga as short as possible so that you can get started quickly.

If you have the time and want to learn something more about the background and many advantages of this card set, then read chapter 1 first.

No matter where you continue to read, I hope you really enjoy putting together your very own series of exercises exactly attuned to your needs and desires. I also hope you experience much joy and enthusiasm in practicing. Working with the cards should increase your well-being and inner resilience, and bring much light and grace into your life.

Best wishes,

Gertrud Hirschi

GERTRUD HIRSCHI

1

THE ADVANTAGES OF THIS YOGA CARD SET

Boundless Possibilities

A deck of yoga cards can entice us to mix, arrange, and combine yoga exercises in new ways. I've worked out a system for using the yoga cards that helps both beginning and advanced students create a practice series that is both meaningful and effective, as well as being kind to the back, and holistic in its approach. This is why the cards have been classified by color and number. Since I love colors, it was easy to come up with the idea of creating the exercise sequences with the help of colors. The more I thought about it, the more sensible, even ingenious, I found the idea to be, since this color sequence primarily corresponds with the colors of the rainbow, or the refractive light in crystal quartz. Color reveals itself in a law of nature when the elements of fire, water, and air combine—to celebrate a marriage, so to speak—for they always create joyful excitement in human beings. Second, the color codes correspond with the color classification of the chakras. Third, the resulting exercise sequence concurs with the principles of color therapy: every color has a healing effect on a specific area of the body and the individual organs, glands, etc. Today most people recognize that colors influence the body as well as the mind and the soul. Here is a brief overview:

Red promotes circulation, makes the body permeable, warms it, and has a stimulating effect on every organ and gland. Red sharpens the sensory organs and fires us up on the mental level. We also want to get things moving with the *warm-up exercises* on the red cards. We want to get warm, release tensions and restlessness, and let spent energy flow away.

Orange is the color of sensuality and joy; it activates the sexual organs. The chakra corresponding to this color is located in the abdomen beneath the navel. The *side bends* also have an effect from the armpits to deep inside the pelvis. They promote permeability, and therefore health, in the area of the sexual organs.

Yellow is particularly effective in the region of the stomach, liver (people suffering from a liver disorder have a yellow cast in the eyes and yellowish skin), gallbladder, and pancreas. Yellow stimulates digestion. The *twisting exercises* on the yellow cards also have their primary effect in this area. Yellow gets a tired mind going again and promotes a light, elated mood.

Green is the chakra color of the heart, and the chest area is primarily affect-ed and opened by *back bends*. Green has a calming effect on the outside, but simultaneously builds up inner strength that a "courageous" person pur-posefully uses to accomplish things that appear to be impossible (like the green sprout that breaks open the hard ground in order to grow and fulfill its purpose in life).

Blue has an effect on the nerve cells, brain, and spinal cord. It corresponds with the *forward bends*, which help stretch the back and neck. Blue is the color of self-communion, silence, loyalty, longing, a sense of security and expansiveness, and sweet melancholy.

Violet is the color of transformation, change, magic, and sorcery. It connects the material world with the spiritual world. The *reverse positions* on the vio-let cards also appeal to these two levels in a special way. This is symbolic of an individual who goes into the depths in order to raise up the treasure of the Utmost.

Brown represents stability and a sense of security. Every meditation posture should be stable and solid, so that lightness can develop in both mind and soul.

White cards contain the balance exercises. They are directed to the entire body. They symbolize the duality from which every body cell, every thought, and every feeling is created—the fundamental level of existence. Any color can develop from this. Every other color is also contained within the color white—all in one and one in all.

I love *black*! However, I've never been able to just wear black—it needs a splash of color. Just as black lets other colors appear stronger, and the value of a number increases when we add a zero to it, the relaxation position, classified with the color black and the number zero, also multiplies the effects of entire practice series at the end of the exercise sequence. This last card symbolizes death and birth—the gateway to a new life, to a new level of life, or perception. After a successful hour of yoga, we also feel as if we've been reborn.

With these few suggestions I've only pointed out the tip of a giant and mysterious iceberg that still remains to be explored. I could also talk about correlations to numerology, but that would go beyond the scope of this work. It is exciting to know that the laws of life are closely connected with each other, and that they support each other, and thereby keep evolution—or our inner growth—in motion.

These cards will help you put together a practice sequence according to a simple system that is completely in keeping with your own needs. You can try out new sequences time and again by interchanging individual exercises or interchanging all the exercises. There are no limits to the possibilities. You will become increasingly certain about feeling what's best for you and for your body. At some point, you will finally be certain: this is right, and this is good for your body in any case.

Brevity is the Soul of Wit!

Since there isn't much room on the cards to describe the exercises, I've used very brief descriptions, concentrating on the essential aspects of each position. This is naturally good for you since you can easily remember the instructions before the exercise and look them up more quickly during the exercise.

Careful Selection of Exercises

I've adhered to the body postures of classic yoga in the selection of exercises. Even the hatha yoga *Pradipika*, one of the oldest yoga writings, speaks of 84 positions. However, very few of these are actually described, and by no means can all these exercises be done, unless you've been doing yoga since you were a small child. This set also consists of 84 cards. I've excluded exercises that should only be done under the direction of an established and/or trained yoga teacher. This means that you shouldn't hesitate to do any of these exercises without a teacher, provided that you take to heart the advice on pages 29–30.

The classic positions are precious and unique because they have a specific and subtle effect on the center of the body (such as the spinal column). Everything you do depends on this area—on every level. The exercises will arouse the basic vital power in the pelvic floor, create the preconditions for it to unfold, and will help fill the mind and heart in order to ultimately connect with cosmic consciousness on the spiritual level. This is also the actual goal of hatha yoga.

The additional effects that occur "incidentally" aren't strange or disconcerting—the flow within the ganglions and nerve paths, their meridians, the lymph channels, and the bloodstream is influenced in a beneficial manner; the musculature of the pelvis, abdomen, chest, shoulders, and back is invigorated and relaxed; the legs and arms, feet and hands are strengthened! All of this determines your health, your feeling of well-being, your moods, and even has a substantial effect on your spiritual development.

I've only selected positions that people with "normal flexibility" can do, with effects that can be directly experienced. These simple, easy-to-do positions in particular fascinate me because of their deep and quick effectiveness. As you practice these exercises you will immediately—and not just at some point in the distant future—sense a feeling of well-being, greater agility, relaxation, and lightness. If this effect doesn't occur at some point, the exercises were probably done too quickly, the pauses for rest between the exercises weren't observed, or the resting position at the end of the exercises was forgotten. The effect can also be lacking if you concentrate too little on the exercises, get lost in negative thoughts, or mull over problems while doing them.

Everything at a Glance

One further advantage of this yoga card set is that you can comprehend an exercise and all the related important information at a glance. You'll see the posture you would like to assume, its static and dynamic nature, and its effect on the body, mind, and soul.

Most of the exercises presented here are *static* in nature. This means that you stay in them for a number of breaths, remaining absolutely still and silent, directing your consciousness to the stretch or to the center of the body (abdomen, chest, or back), while observing your breathing.

Many exercises can also be done *dynamically* by moving one or more body parts to the rhythm of your breathing. In the dynamic variations, you have plenty of leeway, and you will certainly enjoy making full use of these possibilities. If you live in the colder latitudes, these exercises are particularly valuable since the lower temperatures and stress of everyday life seem to indicate a much greater tendency toward tensions than if you live in warmer countries.

The *physical effect* of each position is shown on each card. I don't refer to individual health disorders, such as leukorrhea, kidney stones, etc., because it would be quite controversial. Yoga primarily has a prophylactic effect. It keeps people healthy up to an old age. Everyone has weak spots, or organs that don't work at their best (which means that an organ may function inadequately because it isn't supplied enough blood, or it works too much because the autonomic nervous system is out of balance because of stress, for example). With yoga, we can bring positive energy to individual areas that need strengthening. We release muscle tension and thereby improve circulation, the nerve paths, the meridians. We can support our power of regeneration and healing. The subtle energies are also positively influenced, which means that we may be able to eliminate the cause of physical suffering. An appropriate comparison would be that the body is the landscape, the mind and the feelings are the inhabitants—and we can make it either a paradise or a battlefield.

Many people hope to achieve a great body by doing yoga exercises. Unfortunately, I know from experience that this may not happen. If your body is strong, agile, and well-formed, your mind calm and clear, your heart kind and loving, and your charisma enchants the world around you, then your desire for a great figure will no longer be an issue. You will love your body for what it is.

You will learn more about mental and emotional effects in chapter 3.

2

HOW TO STRUCTURE
AN EXERCISE SERIES

This is quite simple: sort the cards according to the colors and numbers and put them in piles in front of you. You will now have one pile each of red, orange, yellow, green, blue, violet, brown, and white cards, and one single black card. The cards are color-coded to show the following:

1) Red—Warm-Up Exercises;

2) Orange—Side Bends;

3) Yellow—Twists;

4) Green—Back Bends;

5) Blue—Forward Bends;

6) Violet—Inverted Postures;

7) Brown—Sitting Postures;

0) Black—Relaxation Position;

–) White—Balance Exercises.

Select one card from each pile of *numbered* cards and put these in a row according to the numerical order: 1, 2, 3, 4, 5, 6, 7; then add the 0 to them.

Now look at your practice series and think about whether the individual exercises also fit together. Is the sequence of the exercises harmonious? If, for example, you have chosen to be on your abdomen at the beginning, but have to get up for the next exercise, then get back to the prone position for the next exercise, which is followed by one in the long sitting posture—this naturally isn't a harmonious sequence. The transition from one exercise to the next should be appropriate, which means it should take place without too much physical exertion. You can do the first three exercises while standing, the next from a kneestand, two from a prone position, then the diamond posture, and then the relaxation position. You can easily go from the heights to the depths in this way. One exercise flows into the next. If, for example, the yellow card (3) doesn't fit, then simply look for a more appropriate one in the yellow pile; if the green card doesn't fit, then exchange it for another green card, etc.

You will also notice that you have a pile of white cards *without numbers.* These are the balance exercises. Select one card from this pile and add it— like a joker to the series—wherever it fits best according to the aspects mentioned above. The sequence created in this way is largely identical with the classical practice sequences of the great yoga masters.

The examples that follow on pages 11 through 13 show how your series may look.

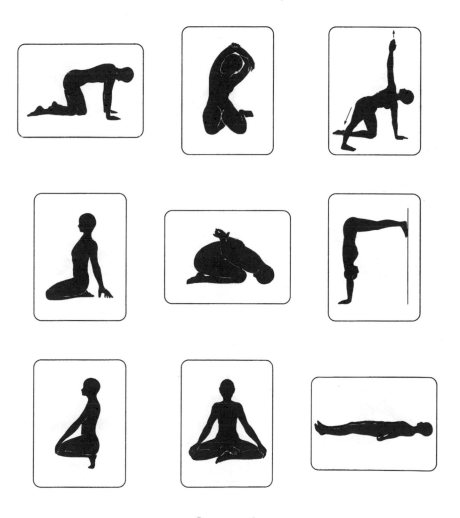

Sequence A

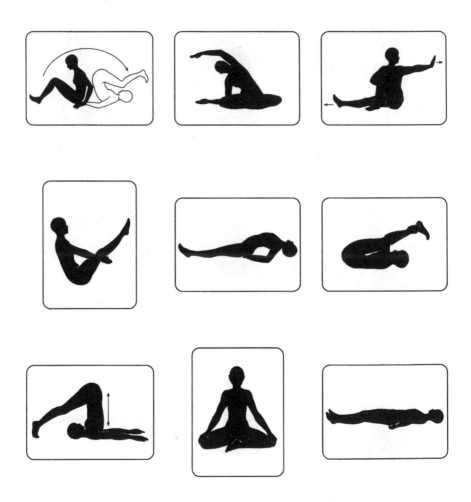

Sequence B

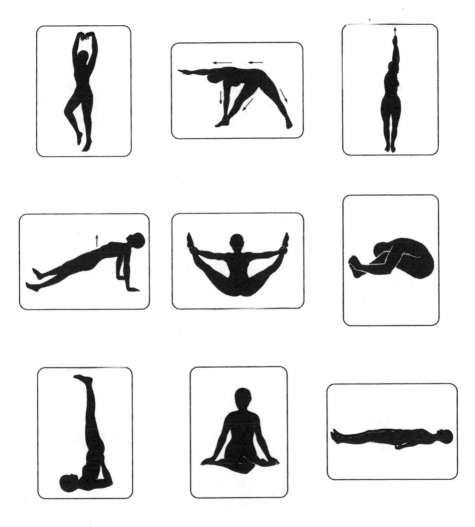

Sequence C

Please don't view this system too narrowly. You can change once from a standing to a prone or supine position, but the body shouldn't have to be reorganized after every exercise. When you move your body into a new position, it is much more work than you may think. If, for example, you observe a very sick or weak person who wants to get up from the floor, or who wants to turn around in bed, you may see how much applied strength is required. You have to use just as much strength as this person may use, but you don't notice it because your body is strong. The movement isn't just a matter of strength alone—a subtle process is also involved. The energy fields within and around you constantly reorganize themselves. *Every hasty movement churns up the energy fields. This consumes energy; in contrast, every slow, harmonious movement calms and harmonizes energy.* Speed mobilizes a great deal of energy within a few seconds, but this energy is quickly spent. Think of a cat that can suddenly jump onto a wardrobe, but who also sleeps almost the entire day; or think of an elephant that constantly has its strength available to it while slowly and steadily taking apart the branches of the trees it eats in the wild.

Yoga is primarily concerned with quieting the body, mind, and soul so that new strength can be built up on every level. The point of these exercises is to create a harmonious sequence in which one exercise flows into the next to bring this repose. If someone complains to me that he or she is missing this peace and harmony in the yoga exercises then I ask about the structure of the practice sequences, since this is usually causing the problem.

Perhaps you don't even want to do a complete practice sequence every day; perhaps *one single exercise* is enough for you—that's wonderful. Then do this in a beautiful, calm, conscious, and slow way—and it is important for you to pause in the *compensation posture for the same amount of time.*

Perhaps you want to do *three exercises* a day—that's wonderful. Then it is best to stay with a series of three, meaning that you select one each from the cards marked 1, 3, and 6.

Perhaps you would like to do *four exercises* a day—that's wonderful. Then it is best to stay with a series of two: 1, 2, 4, and 6.

As you see, you have infinitely many possibilities with this system. Observe the basic rules, let your clear mind and loving heart prevail, and then things are bound to be right!

I should also mention that you shouldn't do a different sequence every day. Put together a practice series and then be loyal to it for a while—several days or even several weeks. As a result, you will become more familiar with the individual exercises, and you can better concentrate on the details, which means experiencing more depth. The body loves repetition and reacts accordingly. Once you are quite familiar with the individual exercises, you must increase your concentration (which will do you good!) so that your thoughts don't drift off and/or you just practice automatically.

After a few days or weeks, exchange one to three of the cards and practice the newly compiled sequence a number of times. Perhaps you can add one exercise that you don't even like. Every posture has an effect on the psychosomatic level, and you can get to know yourself better, particularly in the case of resistance (resistance is the gateway to new territory). Life also becomes interesting when you take a more precise look at your preferences. It is probably clear that you have to bring your sense of humor into play in these acts of self-observation, despite all the required honesty and serious-ness.

In no case should you practice the same sequence for months at a time, because certain muscles are more or less affected with each posture. The stronger one set becomes, the more other muscles will become weak. But you don't want to support some favorites and neglect the others: this is why it is so important to vary the exercises time and again.

Now read the next two chapters, and then you can start practicing.

3

USING BOTH SIDES
OF THE CARDS

On the front of each card you will see a number (except for the white cards), a figure, and a related affirmation. The number refers to the type of exercise (see list on page 9). On the reverse side of the card, you will find the instructions with important information.

Practicing with the Front Side

Before you start exercising, look at the figure on this side for a while and let it have an effect on you. Even this concentrated observation causes your body to adjust to something that seems strange to it at first. This is like having someone demonstrate the position for you.

Now read the affirmation, the positive guiding thought, and meditate a little while on it. Does it appeal to you? Is it right for you, or would you like to change it? How would you like to have it? If necessary, make a note of the new version. The affirmations aren't a must, but can be used as an unexpected opportunity. Slowly repeat the respective sentence one to three times in your breathing rhythm before you assume the posture, or while you pause in the position. Affirmations serve to help you concentrate and achieve self-realization. Just using one to three affirmations per sequence may be enough. Take your choice! Perhaps you are indifferent to the affirmations and prefer to concentrate on your breathing instead. Then practice in this manner.

Practicing with the Reverse Side

Starting Position

If you assume the starting position exactly as described, then you're already well on your way.

Static

A great many of the exercises can be practiced in a static and/or dynamic manner (read about this on page 6 as well); the black figures refer to the static version. What is actually better—static or dynamic? Both versions have their complete justification. The static approach gives more repose and stability; it places demands on you, and promotes concentration. The dynamic approach will relax you, limber you up, making things supple and permeable. It is advantageous to alternate between both variations: a dynamic one follows a static one, etc.

I describe the simplest way to get into the postures as precisely as possible, how long you should stay in the posture, and how you can return to the starting position.

If you stay in a posture for a somewhat longer period of time, you should be sure to let go of any unnecessary tension. Your posture should be steadfast and stable, as well as light and pleasant. Don't be cramped and don't struggle!

In each of the positions, it is important to pay attention to where your thoughts are taking you, and what you are thinking. *The position can be beneficial or harmful to you—it all depends on the quality of your thoughts.* If you practice during a stressful or worrisome time, then you should use the affirmations and direct your thoughts back to these positive guiding words time and again. You will also discover that all the possible kinds of negative thoughts will overcome you during the rest phases—and these are the most important ones when practicing.

Also think about the meaning of the affirmations on the cards, so that the repetitions don't just become automatic babbling. If you are peaceful and centered, you can direct your consciousness to the area of the body being stretched or pressed. Become immersed in your breathing rhythm; with some practice, it can also be felt directly, or as a vibration down into the tips of your toes or fingers. The conscious perception of body areas causes them to be supplied with more energy. This increased energy sparks liveliness, warmth, better circulation, strength, relaxation, regeneration, and healing.

Let's assume that you have difficulties with the right knee or the left shoulder. It wouldn't be sensible to direct your attention to either the right knee or the left shoulder for half an hour and make a habit of this. Every

therapeutic measure contains an imbalance. Let this type of one-sided exercising be the exception. Both sides require increased energy: the sick or weak
side so that it can be healed; and the healthy side because it has more
demands placed on it, meaning that it needs the energy for two.

When you practice holistically, you should generally do this in the following way:

• During the warm-up exercises (1), consciously limber up your face, shoulders, arms, hands, pelvis, legs, and feet.

• During the side bends (2), breathe into the respectively stretched or pressed
side of the body, and consciously perceive it.

• During the twisting (3), breathe into the center of the body (abdomen, or
into the front and back area of the chest), and consciously perceive these
regions.

• During the back bends (4), breathe into the area of the breastbone and/or
the shoulder blades, and consciously perceive this region.

• During the forward bends (5), breathe into the region of the stomach, lum-
bar vertebra, or pelvis, and consciously perceive the respective area.

• During the reverse positions (6), breathe into the head or pelvic region, and
consciously perceive the respective area.

• During the sitting postures (7), direct your consciousness through the
spinal column, from top to bottom when exhaling and from bottom to top
when inhaling.

• During the relaxation position (0), consciously feel the raising and lowering of the chest and abdomen in the breathing rhythm.

• During the balance exercises, keep your eyes fixed on a point and concentrate on the part of the body that keeps you in equilibrium.

You may now feel overtaxed and may wonder how you can keep track of all this. Go slowly and systematically. Direct your attention to the parts of the body that are to bend or twist (see pages 20–21) during the first practice day, to the side bend and twist during the second exercise day, to the back bends and forward bends, and to the inverted position on the third day. The system will then already have become "your second nature." Since everything is also quite logical as well, it will be easier for you to remember it all.

It is also important to spend the same amount of time in the posture on each side for asymmetrical exercises. You can't depend on your feeling since things often work less well on one side than the other; if you practice with the "less comfortable" side, the length of time will seem longer to you. So it's best to get used to counting breaths from the start, since this solves the problem on its own.

One agreeable way to count breaths is done like this: think ONE while inhaling, then OM while exhaling; inhale TWO, exhale OM, etc. This way of counting has a calming and meditative effect. The great yoga masters are very precise about the evenness of asymmetrical exercises. Some time ago I became acquainted with one who even worked with a stopwatch. We should know that the body is a precision instrument par excellence and also reacts accordingly. If we want to find a sense of being centered, harmony, and peace—from which new strength will develop—then we must be aware that only practicing in a harmonious, balanced way will create these qualities.

Optimal

When you pay attention to this section, you can improve the effects of the individual positions several times over. Then you will also practice in a way that does justice to your back and/or can protect you from harm, particularly when you also observe the instructions under the section Compensation Exercises (see pages 23–24).

Dynamic Variations

I often suggest several dynamic variations. *Select just one of them, and do the movement at least eight times.* Too many different movements would bring unrest into your sequence, and that would be unfortunate.

Be sure to start the movements with the same side, if at all possible. Remember, you will only achieve harmony and equilibrium through even, rhythmic, and balanced practicing on both sides.

Alternate between the static and dynamic exercises. This will make your practice time-absorbing, diversified, and the body will oscillate between building up tension and releasing tension. As a result, the tension tonicity that plays an important role in every muscle, every vessel, the ligaments, and every organ, is brought into balance.

Compensation Exercises

These are also very important! Generally, the musculature is twisted in a one-sided manner during side bends and side twists, and the body of the vertebra, including the intervertebral disks, are no longer located on top of each other in an optimal way (even if both sides have been evenly exercised).

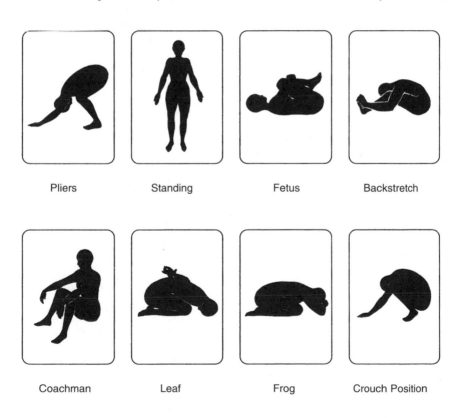

Pliers	Standing	Fetus	Backstretch
Coachman	Leaf	Frog	Crouch Position

Compensation postures

During a forward bend—forward bends are also considered compensation exercises—everything is balanced once again. When you do twists and back bends, the spinal processes are pushed into each other; here as well, the compensation exercise once again creates the necessary distance and reinstates the natural order in the vertebral joints and the many muscles and ligaments along the spinal column. This is the basic rule:

• Every back bend (4), twist (3), and side bend (2) is to be followed by a forward bend (5).

• Ideally, you should remain in the compensation positions for about 10 to 20 breaths. Observe your breathing in the regions of the stomach, back, abdomen, or breastbone.

The most important compensation postures are shown on page 23.

Effect

Physical: As I already mentioned in chapter 2, I don't offer any exercises to heal specific health disorders or that will build the perfect body. However, yoga can help create positive preconditions so that the body will remain healthy, flexible, and strong, so that more energy—either to regenerate or heal, if necessary—is directed into the weak spots. At the same time, the various bodily functions can be brought back into equilibrium. The nadis (subtle energy paths), meridians, nerve paths, lymph channels, and the bloodstream once again become permeable, and every organ and gland can fully perform its activities. If you primarily eat a healthy diet and drink enough liquids, yoga will also support inner cleansing.

When you find the kidneys, head, and hip joint listed in this section, you can assume that these areas are relaxed, calmed, and/or cleansed, which means they have better blood circulation and are supplied with energy, and that the metabolism is activated. I like to compare the body with time-honored, hand-knit socks. These socks are wonderfully soft and pleasant; they protect the feet and keep them warm. In earlier times, the socks were washed once a week, and we should also do yoga at least once a week. The socks were first soaked (warm-up exercises), then pressed in the water and pulled apart again (side bends, forward bends, and back bends). Particularly as a result of pressing them and pulling them apart again, they were rinsed by the water. Dirt and sweat were released and washed away. Exactly the same thing happens in the body. At the end, the socks are wrung out lightly (twists) and hung up at the tips (inverted posture). It is probably clear that we now wash the socks every day, so that we feel good in them; and that the daily practice of yoga is advantageous for well-being and health. It makes sense that the socks must be washed carefully and we should treat our bodies with the same care. Well—there's probably nothing else to be said about it.

Mental-Emotional: Although I'm aware that the following advice is often misunderstood, I would like to mention it anyway, since I know that it can also have many good effects and facilitate and enrich life with yourself and with others. Many people dismiss these "lovely promises," and others in turn are too gullible and think if they are well-behaved and assume some "mysterious" body postures every day, all the problems of everyday life will solve themselves. Both approaches are incorrect. The great "both/and" also applies here. Negative thoughts and feelings, for example, create tensions that can lead to the weak functioning or hyper-functioning of the individual organs. On the other hand, tensions and poorly functioning organs cause unpleasant or burdensome feelings and negative thoughts. This is why we do such things as pulling up our shoulders when we're afraid. If we experience a longer period of time filled with fear, the drawn-up shoulders can become a constant posture. This posture itself can then trigger feelings of fear.

Another example is that people who are afraid of the future often suffer simultaneously from problems with the hip joints—they don't know how things will continue on, etc. Perhaps you are now thinking: "That's not true. I have my shoulder tension because I work at the computer all day long." Or: "My hip problems come from attrition and deposits." These are all consequences, but they don't have to be the causes. If this were true, for example, if the work at the computer or the attrition and deposits were the causes, then all people who work at the computer or have attrition and deposits would then be suffering from the same symptoms. Be that as it may, these causes can be eliminated, or this vicious circle (fears create tensions or tensions create fears) can actually be broken with bodywork that has a relaxing and strengthening effect that improves the posture. The proper attitude toward life also helps.

Many positions also include a look within; this can create clarity and/or improve your attitude toward yourself and your environment. On the other hand, there are other positions that strengthen the body, and this strength is naturally also imparted to the mind and soul. The stronger you feel (physically, mentally, and emotionally), the easier the challenges that life gives you will appear. Wishes and the power of the imagination also influence the bodily functions.

• Meditate on the effects shown and on your own wishes.

• Observe your posture while walking, standing, and sitting. Analyze your actions and reactions in this sense.

• Pay attention to your spoken words and your secret expectations—most of what we believe and talk ourselves into becomes true.

Get to know yourself better; then you can always reorient yourself so that you stay on your own path, or take a new one that you find enjoyable—one that brings you peace, and has a divine goal. The great yoga masters teach that suffering is the result when a person gets on the wrong track.

Everything in my life has really taken a positive turn with yoga. My health, as well as my posture, has improved (I no longer pull my shoulders up to my ears). I've been able to extensively reduce my fears and a tendency to engage in endless, useless brooding; my moods are balanced, and I can again feel joy and peace. If I get out of balance (which naturally can still happen to me today), I can catch myself within a very short time. Moreover, I can always fall back on an inner reservoir of strength when there are unusual tasks to master.

I sincerely wish you the same, but I don't even have to wish it for you since it will happen if you practice yoga on a regular basis—and this is as certain as one and one makes two.

I'd like to make one important comment in closing: It is not the length of the practice time that's decisive, but the intensity, the regularity, and the inner attitude. Practice in a calm, patient way without any specific expectations. Then you will experience wonders.

Make the practice time into the most beautiful minutes of your day. Select a quiet place, a blanket, and appropriate clothing especially for this purpose. Make a ritual of it. Give the whole thing a special framework (music, colors, fragrances, candlelight, etc.). Pamper yourself—then you will also be willing to accept the wonderful gift of practicing.

Now you know the most significant things for the successful practice of yoga, and the following summary will show you what's important in brief. In chapters 4, 5, 6, 7, and 8 you will become familiar with techniques that will help you intensify the effects of the individual exercises.

4

SEVEN GOLDEN RULES AND PRECAUTIONS

Seven Golden Rules

Read the "seven golden rules" until they become second nature for you. You will then get the best out of even a few minutes of bodywork.

1) Focus yourself before you start practicing. Look at the figure on the card for a while; read the instructions carefully; and then think about how you can get into the position with just a few specific movements.

2) Always breathe in through your nose. When you take a posture, remain or move in it, or finish it; your breathing should always be slow, regular, flowing, and fine.

3) Do the warm-up exercises until you are completely limber and warm.

4) Do all the movements in a way that is conscious, flowing, slow, and adapted to your breathing rhythm.

5) While pausing in a position, let go of any unnecessary tension; should uneasy feelings or even pain occur, immediately end the position.

6) In asymmetrical exercises, practice just as long with the other side.

7) Adhere to the necessary pauses for rest between exercises and after the entire bodywork. This will multiply the effect of the whole.

Precautions

Please observe the following rules as well:

• At least two hours should pass after a meal before you start with the exercises.

• This card set has been created for people who are healthy.

• Do not do any of the exercises if you have an acute flu, acute backache, inner inflammation, injuries of any type, unstable blood pressure, and following operations.

• Do not assume any inverted positions during menstruation.

• During pregnancy, please consult a doctor and/or a yoga teacher specially trained for this situation.

• *In case of doubt, always consult a doctor.*

5

THE PRANAYAMA
TECHNIQUE

The pranayama exercises—special breathing techniques—are an important component of classical yoga. In English, *pranayama* means control or expansion of the vital energy. The following exercises will help you control your breathing so that it can optimally fulfill its function; and this creates beneficial conditions to allow the vital energy to unfold. You can imagine this process to be something like a fire that quietly smolders and smokes when the stove and chimney aren't cleaned, or the fire isn't supplied with enough oxygen. The same fire is full of energy, and radiates warmth and light when properly fanned.

The yogis teach that the way a person breathes is the way he or she is— this is how the person thinks, feels, what his or her moods are like, how this person lies down, sits, stands, and acts. The sentence can also be turned around: The way a person thinks, feels, lies, stands . . . is how he or she breathes. This means that regulation of breathing also regulates bodily functions, posture, thinking, feeling, and moods. In short, it can decisively influence the entire quality of life.

This means that how well we feel, how healthy we are, how clearly we think, and how productive we are is largely dependent on our breathing. With the following exercises we can once again find our individual breathing rhythm that optimally supplies us with energy on the one hand, and positively influences our moods and feelings on the other. At the same time, our concentration and every other function of the brain is improved.

> The quality of the breath is best when it is rhythmical, slow, flowing, and fine. Then the largest amount of prana (vital energy) streams in, and then it best circulates through the body or its energy fields. The quality of the breath decisively influences the autonomous nervous system and therefore also every bodily function associated with it. It strengthens the mind, which improves the mood, and activates every type of cerebration.

I have selected some exercises for you that have benefited me personally. You can practice these alone without difficulty. The effect of breathing is tremendous in both the positive and the negative sense. This means you should always practice to a sensible extent—carefully and gently.

Before you start with the breathing exercises, you should first become conscious about *how* your breathing is; second, *where* your breathing areas are; and third, how you can maintain your *own rhythm* for a while. Just becoming aware of this already has a balancing and regenerating effect.

Three-Part Breathing

By doing the *three-part breathing exercises*, you will become aware of the quality of your breathing. You observe how the air streams in, the small pause during the fullness of breath, how the air streams back out again, and the small pause when the lungs are empty. *Let your breath become slow—rhythmic flowing and fine. Breathe consciously and immediately let go of any other thoughts.* If you practice regularly (about 10 minutes a day), this way of breathing will be carried into everyday life, and as a result, you will automatically take in more oxygen and vital energy, making you more vital on every level.

So now lie down on your back, and place your hands on your abdomen as shown in the illustration below. Then observe how the abdominal wall rises when you inhale and sinks again when you exhale. If this isn't the case,

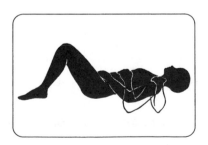

or if you feel the opposite, then press your hands on the abdominal wall during exhalation, and let go of the pressure when inhaling. If this doesn't work either, then ask someone to do this for you (in a very loving way, naturally!). In this manner, with just a few breaths I've been able to teach abdominal breathing to people who haven't been able to do it for years. Breathe this way 10 to 30 times.

Now place your hands on your ribs and observe how the ribs rise during inhalation and sink again during exhalation. If you don't feel anything, then again press the hands on the ribs (as if you wanted to squeeze a concertina) and also let go of the pressure when the air streams in. Practice in this way 10 to 30 breaths.

Now place your fingers on your collarbones, with upper arms resting flat on the ground, and feel your breath in the area of the collarbones. If you don't feel anything, then press your fists against the collarbones until you do—10 to 30 breaths.

Once you have mastered this first exercise, you can even manipulate the rhythm (but gently!). *If you desire more peace in your head, heart, and body, slow down and intensify your exhalation. But if you want more élan and a feeling of freshness, slow down and intensify the inhalation.* Ten breaths may be enough—then return to your normal breathing rhythm.

The Complete Yoga Breath

With the yogic breathing, you can "seal" the three-part breathing. During inhalation, first swell your abdomen, then your chest, and finally the upper lung region. Hold your breath for three seconds, and while exhaling slightly draw in the abdominal wall, lowering the chest area and shoulders. Then wait attentively until the impulse for the next breath occurs—and the game starts over again; 3 to 10 breaths are adequate.

Alternate Nostril Breath

If you desire a better sense of physical balance and serenity in thinking and feeling, or more equilibrium in your moods, then the *alternate nostril breath* (Sanskrit: *nadi sodhana*; English: "purification of the subtle energy paths") will help. Always be sure that both your nostrils are free, because if you inhale and exhale too much on the right or left side this will cause your nervous system, which influences every physical function, to become unbalanced. The first variation cleans the nasal passages, thereby creating favorable conditions for the following variations. For all three, assume a centered, upright sitting posture, and by moving your hands—one points down to the ground and the other points upward—bring the earth energy into harmony with the heavenly energy (yin and yang).

Alternate Nostril Breath I

Assume the Meditation Posture, straighten your back, and keep your neck erect. Close the right nostril with your right thumb (the fingers of the left hand have contact with the floor), and then inhale and exhale through the left nostril. Then close the left nostril with the left thumb, and inhale and exhale through the right nostril. If the nasal passages aren't completely open at the start, then blow out strongly through them (like a snorting horse). Let your breathing become slow, flowing, and fine.

- Inhale and exhale 7 times through the left nostril.

- Inhale and exhale 7 times through the right nostril.

- Breathe 3 times through both nostrils.

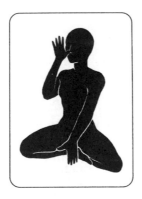

Alternate Nostril Breath II

- Close the left nostril, inhale and exhale on the right side.

- Close the right nostril, inhale and exhale on the left side.

- Repeat by alternating 6 to 12 times, and then

- Slowly inhale and exhale 3 times through both nostrils.

Alternate Nostril Breath III

- Close the right nostril and inhale on the left side.

- Now close the left nostril and exhale on the right side.

- Repeat by alternating 6 to 12 times, and then

- Slowly inhale and exhale 3 times through both nostrils.

Once you have a good mastery of these three variations, you can intensify the effect even more by lengthening somewhat the pauses after the inhalation and/or exhalation. While you do this, count: one—OM, two—OM, three—OM.

Chin Press (Murcha-Pranayama)

This breathing exercise can trigger a heady feeling and create a wondrous inner peace. This may mean a pleasant retreat from the outer world, which sometimes feels very good when a person is too entangled in it. According to Yesudian, a great yoga master, this exercise also strengthens the willpower and powers of resistance.

Assume the Meditation or Diamond Posture.

- Inhale deeply.

- Hold your breath, lower your head, and press your chin onto your breastbone.

- Remain in this position for 3 to 7 seconds.

- Raise your head and slowly let the air stream out.

- Repeat 7 times.

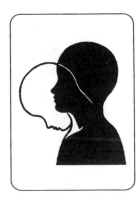

HA Breath

It's great to "let off steam" with this exercise. When you throw yourself forward with a powerful "HA"—while exhaling through your mouth—you can get rid of a great deal of bottled-up and spent energy. This happens not only in the body, but also in the soul and mind.

Stand with your legs apart, throw your arms upward while inhaling, and then bend forward while exhaling with a powerful "HA" (as if you were chopping wood with an ax). Your entire body will vibrate along with this movement. It's enough to do it 5 to 10 times. Be sure that you bend your knees well when you throw yourself forward, and that your back and neck don't get into a back bend position when you swing back up again.

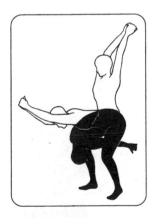

Cooling Breath (Sitali)

This exercise works against an entire range of stomach problems and accelerates the elimination of toxins (poisons). It therefore has a cleansing effect. When someone is hot-headed, it also has a cooling and calming effect.

Assume the Meditation or Diamond Posture—straighten your back. Hold your tongue in the shape of a pipe between your lips. Slowly inhale through the pipe-shaped tongue, close your mouth, and hold your breath (up to 10 seconds). Then exhale through the nose in a slow and relaxed way. Repeat 5 to 10 times.

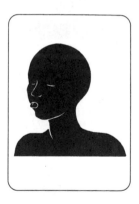

Hissing Breath (Sitkari)

This exercise also has a cleansing effect, particularly in the area of the throat and larynx. In addition, it synchronizes the right and left hemispheres of the brain and stimulates certain meridians through the contact between the tongue and roof of the mouth.

Assume the Meditation or Diamond Posture—straighten your back. Place the tip of your tongue on the roof of your mouth and inhale. Close your mouth, hold your breath for a few seconds, and then slowly exhale. Repeat 5 to 10 times.

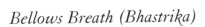

Bellows Breath (Bhastrika)

A great deal of oxygen is taken in and much carbon dioxide is eliminated in this breathing exercise. The movement of the abdominal wall massages the liver, spleen, kidneys, and pancreas, activating their functions and promoting digestion. This trains lung tissue and the diaphragm. It also strengthens the nervous system, stimulates the brain, and refreshes the entire body.

Assume the Meditation or Diamond Posture—straighten your back and place your hands on your abdomen.

- Inhale deeply.

- Exhale well.

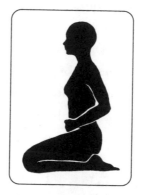

- With the full use of the abdominal wall, now vigorously suck in and expel the air several times as if with a bellows. Do this 5 to 10 times.

- When concluding the exercise, exhale vigorously one more time.

- Now finish with several slow, calm breaths. Repeat 3 times.

Shining Head (Kapalabhati)

Here's one more exercise in closing. This will wake you up, give you a clear, cool, and light head, and lift your spirits. It detoxifies, since much spent air is expelled, stimulates the digestion, trains the abdominal musculature, and cleanses the nasal passages and maxillary sinuses.

Assume the Meditation or Diamond Posture—straighten your back and place your hands on your thighs.

Vigorously blow out the air through the nose (as if you had something in it that has to get out). You will notice that your abdominal wall helps you do this. So now make conscious use of your abdominal wall: pull it in with a jerking motion and then let go again. Do these jerks quickly and make the sound of a snorting steam locomotive. Direct your consciousness at your nose and forehead while you do this. After 10 to 20 of these exhalations, once again breathe in a calm, slow, and fine way.

Where and When Should You Practice Pranayama?

When the weather is warm and mild, you can practice pranayama out in the open countryside; otherwise, do it in a warm, well-aired room.

These exercises naturally work best if you do them on a regular basis. You can reserve a special time for them in the evening or morning (3 to 15 minutes) or integrate them with the bodywork. Select just one to three from the different variations and practice these for a while. Then change them again. Yesudian always put pranayama at the beginning of the hour, and other yoga masters practice them at the close of the hour. I like to do these exercises after the inverted positions, before the meditation.*

---

*Perhaps you are already familiar with pranayama techniques, but have learned these in a different way in part. Don't be confused—pranayama isn't practiced in exactly the same way by all the schools. Choose the version that's best for you.

6

THE MENTAL PATH
OF YOGA

The most important cards in this set are the brown cards (7). On these cards are the sitting postures, which are to be assumed for several minutes after the bodywork. With them, we take the mental path of yoga—the royal path of yoga, as the old masters called it.

"Mental" means our thinking—our habits of thought that we consciously perceive in the silence of sitting and, if necessary, that can be changed. We should be aware that our health, our moods, and our entire life is directly or indirectly dependent on our thoughts. It is worth it to give consideration to the process of thinking at some point. It is worth it to observe how you think. It is worth it to change habits of thought that bring suffering.

"Clear thinking" is often mentioned in yoga. I like to differentiate between *clear* and *cloudy thoughts.* When the air is clear—without cloud formations—the sky is blue, the sun shines, and our vital spirits are awake. When it is foggy and cloudy, the effort of getting into better spirits is usually greater—except for when a person is head over heels in love, or decides to spend the cloudy day in bed with a good book. We can also lose ourselves in *clear* or *cloudy* thoughts, and our moods will follow accordingly. Pondering about worries, past suffering, or fears about the future doesn't make this all go away. To the contrary—it fuels these concerns with new energy and afflicts us even more. Even Patanjali, who wrote the first and most important pearls of yoga wisdom and rules for behavior, warned about doing this.

In yoga—as in psychology as well—people talk about habitual thinking. Like any other habits, these have been built up over the course of time, or have been assumed from role models. These habits can bring joy or suffering into your life. With increasing self-knowledge—meaning the more you observe and get to know yourself—you can discover and change these habits. Some discipline and patience is required to do this, but it is always worth the effort. Before you can undertake any meaningful changes, it is important to know *how* you think. The following exercises are meditation suggestions that you should repeat frequently at regular intervals during a period of several days or weeks. The length of a session should be about 10 to 20 minutes.

> Observe your breathing. As soon as you think of something
> else, look at this thought from all sides and recognize its quality
> (positive or negative, constructive or depressing, light or cloudy,
> oriented toward memories or the future, necessary or
> unnecessary). Let go of the thought and turn back
> to your breathing again.

At the end, you can take stock of how constructive or depressing the thoughts were that came up, or what type of coloration most of your thoughts had. The second step naturally involves considering how you could change your cloudy thought-structures.

> Observe your breathing. As soon as you think of something
> else, recognize and name this thought. In case it is of a negative
> nature, think about its opposite. Then return to observing your
> breathing. If another thought arises, . . . etc.

In the process of learning yoga, we assume that *thoughts always influence and determine our feelings and moods,* and not the other way around. Exceptions to this are hunger and thirst, food that is too heavy, too little sleep, hurry and stress, a physical sense of unease, and pain. All of these components—except for pain—can be reduced to a minimum by planning our lives in a sensible way.

I like to differentiate between conscious, half-conscious, and unconscious thoughts in this respect. When, for example, you spontaneously ask someone: "What were you thinking of just now?" she can either respond with very clear information (conscious thoughts) or she may just know the vague and general meaning of what she was thinking (half-conscious), or she must admit she doesn't know what she was thinking (unconscious).

The latter, *the unconscious thoughts, are largely responsible for our moods, health, attitude toward life, and our overall way of living.* These thoughts are like magnets that draw everything that we direct them at into our lives. In meditation, when we calm down and observe our thoughts, we can become aware of our unconscious thoughts. We can become conscious of them in the silence and, if necessary, even reverse their polarity, meaning we think about their opposite for a while.

When we know that negative thoughts of every type rob us of strength in the body, mind, and soul, then we are also aware that working on thought structures is of the greatest importance, and should never be neglected.

One further mental help in life that we can experience through yoga is asking questions of our inner self. We should know that we only make use of a small portion of our brain. The large part of it lies fallow—and this part stores a great deal of information—and we aren't even conscious of it. In the silence of meditation we can become conscious of such information or, expressed in other terms: we have a power within us, a higher consciousness, that is not only bound to the present but also understands deeper correlations with the past and has a better perspective of the future. I like to compare the course of our lives with the course of a river: the daytime consciousness stands directly at the river, and its point of view only goes as far as the next bend; the higher consciousness stands on a mountain and has a panoramic view as a result. It sees the course of the river from the source to the mouth. During meditation we can make contact with the higher consciousness, ask it questions, and receive its instructions. We can also ask it for any type of help, both in the large and the smallest matters—and will also receive it if we are willing to contribute our very best. This type of meditation also builds up self-confidence and a trust in God, giving us the true security that we can only find within ourselves.

> Turn within and observe your breathing until you are calm.
> Now imagine a symbol or figure of light for your higher
> consciousness. State your concern in clear words, describe it
> precisely, and ask your question. Now turn to your breathing,
> and listen quietly and patiently within. Be prepared
> to receive an answer or advice.

The answer may come immediately—as a thought, voice, or feeling—or only later in bed, in the shower, while reading a book, or encountering a friend who "coincidentally" says the right thing.

We can also differentiate between *superficial* and *deep thoughts*. Superficial thoughts are like the waves on the surface of the water that are caused by the wind (mind). A person sitting in a boat and rocking on the waves would have to hold tight with all his strength in order not to be thrown into the water. But if the boat is heavy or even has an anchor, then the boat can break the waves or remain anchored until things have calmed down again. The hands are free for taking action, the head for thinking, and the heart—for enjoying.

According to yoga, superficial thoughts are caused by a restless mind. They often bring suffering. Peaceful, deep thoughts dissolve suffering because clarity, trust, and confidence develop. If, for example, someone says something unpleasant to you, such as "You don't have any time for me," or "Your work is inadequate," your superficial reaction to this causes superficial thoughts, and vice versa. This is expressed in insulting or derogatory thoughts, or expressions of them, such as "You're an idiot anyway," in generalizations, such as "Everyone says I'm . . .," or in pessimism, exaggerations, or flights into the past, etc.

However, if you would think about the sentence, "You never have time for me!" for 10 minutes—about each word, the person, the situation, then you would certainly come up with completely different and interesting conclusions. You would react to it in a totally different way.

The following exercise can serve you as an anchor; it can increase your clear vision and bring peace and depth into every personal concern, which is so important for solving problems and conflicts.

Observe your breathing, slow down your exhalation, and
lengthen the pauses between inhalation and exhalation. Now
observe your problem from all sides in a calm and relaxed way.
Direct your consciousness back to your breathing again, and
after a while consider your problem from all sides again.
Go back to breathing, . . . etc.

With the help of this exercise, you can overcome fears and doubts and
work on problems until they are solved. I believe that almost any problem
can be solved in this way, because the core of the solution is always present,
concealed in the depths, like a pearl at the bottom of the ocean.

Don't strive violently for an immediate solution, but end the exercise
after a while and put the matter aside for the time being. It will continue to
thrive in your subconscious mind, and it may well be that the solution is suddenly there—like a bolt out of the blue—in a quiet moment, when you are
completely relaxed. When doing this exercise, be sure that you don't get lost
in persistent pessimism.

Here is one last little exercise that has been the most help to me in cut-
ting down on burdening thoughts and building up edifying, positive ones. I
like to talk about "wishing something for yourself." On the basis of my experience, I now know that wishes tend to be fulfilled. Many of my yoga students have already had wonderful experiences with this. Another example is
that my domestic helper joyfully told me how she found the house she

desired, and the bills that should have ended up being quite high miracu-
lously shrank away or didn't even materialize at all. We are completely jus-
tified in having wishes, if these aren't at the cost of the environment or other
people. We are also permitted to have wishes of a material nature. The wish
for a meaningful job that we enjoy and in which we can apply our talents, or
the desire for a loving relationship, are both certainly realistic. We may also
wish that we increasingly become (in the outside world) what we actually are
within our innermost self—happy, understanding, and loving people. The
greatest desire is always the longing for divine unity—you could call this
universal or cosmic consciousness. People who no longer have any wishes
may be preventing this spiritual development.

> Calm yourself by consciously slowing down your breathing.
> Now think about your wishes. Then express one wish with
> clear words, and repeat it several times to the rhythm of your
> breathing. Promise to do—or stop doing—everything in
> your power so that this wish can be fulfilled. Leave the rest
> to the Divine Being. Give thanks for the divine help,
> and continue to observe your breathing.

You can present a number of wishes, or even worries of any type, in this
way. The Divine Being is a tremendous power and energy. It is more than
willing to help us in concerns both small and large, bringing everything to a
happy ending. It can only bring things to a happy ending. This may even

mean dying, if we have the right attitude (and this is something we can wish for) about it.

We can have great influence on our thinking and the creation of our present and future when using these meditations. One last bit of advice on this topic: *Despite all the seriousness, don't forget your sense of humor!*

7

THE BANDHA
TECHNIQUE

The practice of the three bandhas also belongs to classical yoga. Translated literally, *bandha* means "lock." Specific muscles are tensed during these locking exercises; they are closed. Although I had already been familiar with these exercises for a long time, I've only actually been doing them myself since I read an article in the German magazine *Esotera* (2/96 edition) about a research project within the scope of which the bandha's effect was "coincidentally" discovered. After extensive studies, the researchers came to the conclusion that the tensing of the PC muscle, the pubococcygeus muscle in the perineum between the anus and the genital organs, has the effect of an energy pump on the brain. This energy natural-ly benefits every other bodily function as well, and has a considerable effect on a person's moods and habits of thought. If you practice this bandha on a regular basis, you will basically feel better and have more emotional-mental energy available to you. People who do this feel generally more satisfied and relaxed, are more cheerful and creative, and have better concentration; they have the élan to start something, follow through on it, and also complete it. Moreover, it has been reported that this exercise can extensively improve the quality of meditation as well, increasing the ability to concentrate and creating the necessary peace from which new strength can unfold again. These were reasons enough for me to start with the practice, especially since it is very simple and doesn't take much time.

However, instead of just practicing one bandha, you should do all three. With the *Mula Bandha*, the energy is kindled in the pelvic floor and caused to rise upward. The other two promote the continued climbing of the energy from the pelvis to the head. Do this in the following way:

• Assume the Meditation Posture while sitting with an erect back.

• Now press your hands on your thighs and simultaneously contract the musculature around the perineum by tensing the muscles of the anus and the sphincter of the bladder, as if you wanted to hold back feces and urine. Maintain this tension for several seconds and then slowly let go of all tension. This contraction is called the *Mula Bandha*.

• Now you can pull the abdomen inward and upward at the same time; this is how you practice the *Uddiyana Bandha*.

• If you now also press your chin on your larynx and raise your breastbone, then you are also practicing the third bandha, the *Jalandhara Bandha*.

I mainly practice these bandhas at the beginning of meditation in order to more quickly and deeply get into the meditative state. Repeating them 7 times is often enough for me. When I notice a drop in energy while doing some type of mental work, this technique has the effect of a stimulant for me (particularly if I get up afterward, open the window, and have a good stretch).

The effect is intensified by about 30 percent if you face toward the west while doing it. You can naturally do this little exercise anywhere you like. The important thing about it is to always sit forward on your sitting bones and keep your back straight.

It is actually quite simple!

Sit up straight, contract the PC muscle while inhaling and the abdominal wall will automatically tense—then tense it a bit more. Now pull down your chin and raise your breastbone at the same time. Slowly count to 10 while staying in this position. Now let go of every tension once again and raise your chin. Repeat 3 to 10 times.

8

THE MUDRA
TECHNIQUE

In this chapter, you will learn an additional technique from ancient India that can positively influence the quality of your meditation. Depending on what you want to accomplish with your meditation, you can intensify its effect with a mudra—a specific position of the hand and fingers. I will introduce some mudras of classical yoga that I have practiced myself. I have experienced their pleasant effects. While doing this, I have also discovered that the effect of the side bends and twists is somewhat intensified when I just concentrate on the individual fingers. Don't practice the mudras for more than 15 minutes, since they can have the effect of a strong medication: they heal when properly dosed but an overdose can have negative consequences.

> It is very important that you concentrate completely on your hands and/or fingers (especially the pressure points of the fingers) for a number of breaths.

The Gesture of Meditation (Dhyani Mudra)

If you want to collect your thoughts and achieve peace in order to revitalize yourself, then place your hands into each other like bowls: the left hand in the right hand, the thumbs touching each other. The hands and arms form a closed energy circuit (as shown in the illustration below), which also corresponds to the leg position in the meditation position.

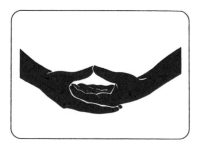

The Gesture of Knowledge (Jnana Mudra)

In yoga, this gesture is considered to be a universal remedy against mental states of tension and disorder; it supports the memory and concentration, as well as relaxing the mind. It also has a spiritual significance that makes it precious to me. The thumb symbolizes cosmic consciousness and the index finger human consciousness. They are united in this gesture.

Position: The tips of the index finger and the thumb lie lightly on top of each other; the rest of the fingers are stretched in a relaxed position.

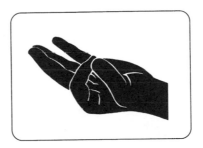

The Gesture of Prayer (Atmanjali Mudra)

This gesture brings harmony, balance and repose, silence and peace. It is also suitable for when a heart's desire is to be fulfilled, such as when you ask the Divine Being for something, thank it for something, or praise it. Furthermore, it synchronizes the right and left hemispheres of the brain. However, if you want to remember something, need a good idea, or are searching for the solution to a problem, then place the fingertips onto each other. This will increase availability of the right hemisphere of the brain as well (memory, creativity, emotion).

Position: Place the palms of the hands together in front of the chest and exercise a light pressure on the breastbone with the thumbs.

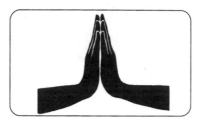

For Collection

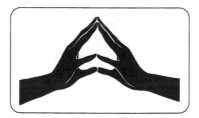

For Concentration

Purification Mudra (Apan Mudra)

The Apan Mudra helps remove waste materials and toxins from the body and cleanses the entire system. If you would like to get rid of old patterns of thought or bad feelings, this mudra—used during a meditation—supports this process.

Position: The tips of the middle finger and ring finger are placed on the tip of the thumb; the rest of the fingers remain stretched.

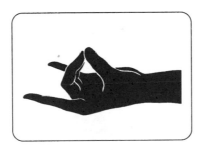

Earth Mudra (Prithvi Mudra)

In India, it is known that this gesture balances a deficit of earth energy in the body, which can cause psychological weakness and diminished vitality. This mudra also gives us both inner and outer equilibrium.

Position: Place the tips of the thumb and ring finger together using light pressure.

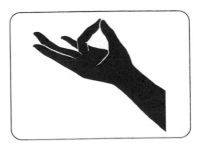

Life Mudra (Prana Mudra)

With the help of this mudra, you can overcome fatigue and nervousness.

Position: Place the tips of the thumb, ring finger, and little finger together; the rest of the fingers remain stretched.

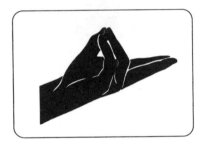

CLOSING REMARKS

Yoga can be connected with any project in a direct and indirect way. We plan something, create an order for it, work out the individual steps, take the path, and deal with every task as it comes up, resolve every challenge that blocks the way, and direct our eyes to the objective time and again. In this process, the mind is completely included, challenged, and supported; the heart—love—comes to fruition, and the most important aspect, the connection with the Divine Being (yoga in completely concrete terms) is constantly renewed, improved, and deepened. Most appropriate are projects that require the very utmost from us and cause us to make renewed appeals for divine help to insure success.

The joy is great when the work is accomplished—when we are allowed to experience how everything fits together, because an energy, a power, is at work. And this power is beyond our ability to comprehend. I hope that all the people who read this book will use the power of yoga to change their lives.

BIBLIOGRAPHY

Desikachar, T. K. *The Heart of Yoga: Developing a Personal Practice*. Rochester, VT: Inner Traditions International, 1995.

————. *Religiousness in Yoga: Lecture on Theory and Practice*. Mary L. Skelton and J. R. Carter eds. Landham, MD: University Press of America, 1980.

Feuerstein, Georg. *The Philosophy of Classical Yoga*. Rochester, VT: Inner Traditions, 1996.

Freedman, Miriam and Janice Hankes. *Yoga at Work*. Shaftesbury, UK: Element, 1996.

Groves, Dawn. *Yoga for Busy People*. Los Altos, CA: New World Library, 1995.

Haich, Elisabeth. *Self Healing, Yoga and Destiny*. Santa Fe, NM: Aurora, 1983.

Kriyananda, Goswami. *The Spiritual Science of Kriya Yoga*. Chicago: Temple of Kriya Yoga, N.D.

Luby, Sue. *Hatha Yoga for Total Health: Handbook of Practical Programs*. New York: Prentice-Hall, 1977.

Mohan, A. G. *Yoga for Body, Breath, & Mind: A Guide to Personal Reintegration*, rev. ed., Kathaleen Miller, ed. Portland, OR: Rudra Press, 1995.

Ohlig, Adelheid. *Luna Yoga: Vital Fertility & Sexuality*. Meret Liebenstein, trans. Woodstock, NY: Ash Tree, 1995.

Saraswati, Swami Janakananda. *Yoga, Tantra and Meditation in Daily Life*. York Beach, ME: Samuel Weiser, 1992.

Yesudian, Selvarajan. *Yoga Week by Week*. D. Q. Stephenson, trans. New York: Routledge Chapman & Hall. 1988.

Yesudian, Selvarajan and Elisabeth Haich. *Yoga & Health*. New York: Routledge Chapman & Hall, 1988.

INDEX

ABOUT THE AUTHOR

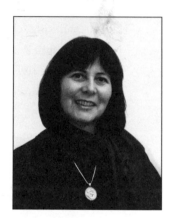

G ertrud Hirschi completed her training to be a
yoga teacher with the professional associa-
tion of German Yoga Teachers. For the past 16
years, she has taught at her own yoga school in
Zurich, and holds seminars in Switzerland,
Germany, and Greece. Gertrud Hirschi is the
author of several other books published in German.